STOP BINGING

*How to stop overeating and
emotional eating.
How to lose weight when you just
can't cut down on food.*

By
Kerry Glennon

TABLE OF CONTENTS

Introduction

Bingeing is a word that used to mean just one thing: excessive drinking. Now, the word is more widely used to refer to overeating. To a lot of people, bingeing is something as inconsequential as a basic overindulgence or a simple dietary lapse. To others, it is a total or partial loss of the control you have over food. This is a bigger problem than most people realize, and it's not a problem only for Western countries. Despite being a problem that affects many people, we still know very little about it.

Is purging always preceded by bingeing? Is this a lifelong health problem? Can it be fixed? Is it a sign of something much worse? How can we tell the difference between a simple overindulgence and true bingeing? What makes a person prone to binge eating? How can I fix it? These are critical questions that most people ask.

The Meaning of the Word 'Binge'

The definition of 'binge' has evolved over the years. It was widely used in the nineteenth century, and it meant 'a heavy drinking spree,' and it remains one of the definitions you will find in the Oxford English Dictionary. The other definitions influenced by modern times include 'overindulgence' or 'overeating.'

According to the eleventh edition of Merriam Webster's Collegiate Dictionary, bingeing is basically an unrestrained indulgence or overindulgence. This indulgence has been reported both by men and women. For some, it starts out as an occasional binge, which remains an occasional binge that has no adverse effect on their lives. For others, it progresses into a significant problem that starts to negatively affect many areas of their lives. The reason a lot of people can't distinguish between the two is their similarities and the lack of information people have on this behavior.

Due to this confusion, research has been conducted into the experiences of binge eaters and while all accounts aren't exactly the same, there are two very distinct features that binge eaters had in common : the amount of food consumed is seen as excessive even by the eater, and they all seem to lose control during the indulgence. So when trying to identify a binge, check if the food being consumed is noticeably more than what others would have under the same circumstances.

Characteristics of a Binge

I read somewhere about a girl that said she would randomly select whatever food she could get her hands on and just stuff her face with it sometimes without even chewing it. After some minutes, she started to feel guilty and scared because her stomach would start to ache, but she wouldn't be able to stop. She complained about a rise in temperature and how she would only be able to stop eating when she felt really sick. Going through personal accounts of binge eating can be a real eye-opener. Let's take a look at certain spot-on traits of a real binge.

Feelings: The first few moments of a binge can feel like heaven. The feeling and taste of the food on your tongue will feel so intense and pleasurable. However, these feelings vanish as quickly as they came and are immediately replaced by feelings of guilt, shame and disgust as you continue to stuff your face uncontrollably. This is very common among binge eaters. They feel repulsed by their actions, yet they continue to eat.

Consumption Speed: Binge eaters are not slow eaters. It is typically a rapid process. They stuff their faces as if on auto-pilot sometimes without even chewing the food. Others push the food down their throats with drinks, particularly sodas, and this is another primary reason they feel full and bloated really quickly. For people with bulimia, drinking a lot makes it easier to throw up later.

Agitation: It's a common habit for binge eaters to wander around or pace their environment while they eat. It's almost like desperation. Some people have described the craving to be some kind of powerful force that makes them eat, and this is the reason compulsive eating and binge eating can be used interchangeably. This isn't the only behavior of agitation they exhibit. Some might go as far as taking food that doesn't belong to them, shoplift or even consume food that has been discarded just to satisfy a craving. Guess what happens right after... Feelings of disgust, degradation and shame.

Allow me to paint a quick picture. You start by having a bowl of oatmeal, which you eat as quickly as you can and move on to have three or four extra bowls. By now, you should know that your control has gone to the dogs, and you're already knee-deep in bingeing but you can't seem to stop. You feel very tense during the desperate search for anything to eat. Anything at all. You run around looking for discarded food even while acknowledging how disgusting that is. Luckily for you, you find some nosh and wolf it down. Sometimes, you decide to go into town to 'check out' stores and do a bit of grocery shopping. And, what if you don't have enough cash on you to buy all the food you want? Some binge eaters resort to shoplifting, which is a Class A misdemeanor.

Trance-like state: Some people have described the binge like the feeling of being stuck in a trance, almost like their behavior is being remotely controlled. If you have had an experience just like this, you understand when I say that it feels like you're not the person that's actually eating.

Some people also claim to engage in some other activity like listening to loud music or reading a book while bingeing because it distracts them from what they're doing, which pretty much prevents them from owning up to their bad habit. I'll paint a picture. You wake up with that feeling in your stomach, maybe someone upset you deeply yesterday, or you're just sad or lonely and you feel this overwhelming urge to binge. Almost immediately, you begin to feel clammy and hot, and then your mind goes dark. You make your way towards the food and dig in quickly, scared that you might start to think and feel guilty if you eat slowly.

You get up and pace. At the same time, you eat or watch a series, anything distracting enough to keep your mind off what you're doing because once you have enough time to think about the fact that you're bingeing, you might even feel sadder because it's a reminder that you have a bad habit. Seem familiar?

Secrets: A typical binge happens in secret because of the shame that is attached to the habit. Some people feel so much shame that drives them to hide it for as long as they can; months and even years. The most basic way they do this is to eat as frequently as possible when in the presence of others. Do you generally eat regular portions during a family meal or when around friends then go back later to swallow all the leftovers? Do you sneak food into your bedroom so you can indulge with zero fear of getting caught? Do you go shopping for food right after work and eat more than half of it in the privacy of your car before you get home?

Doing this reduces any chance of getting help because even with all the disgust and shame you feel afterward, you do it again and again and again because you honestly don't know any other healthy ways of dealing with stress.

Losing Control: Like I mentioned before, losing control is one of the significant features of bingeing. It is what makes regular overeating different from bingeing. This particular characteristic of the habit varies between individuals.

Let's talk about loss of control. Some said they feel it way before the bingeing even starts; others said it slowly builds while they eat, and others said that it kicks in immediately after they realize just how much they have eaten.

An interesting thing to note is that a lot of people who have been bingeing for years claim that the loss of control has diminished over the years because they became comfortable with the fact that their binges are lifelong. So they don't even try to fight the urge anymore.

Others even plan into the future for what they perceive as inevitable binges, which automatically adds some extra cushion to their comfy chair of bad habits. Still, on the plus side, this method gives them a certain amount of control over where the binges happen and availability of food thus saving them from a lot of uncomfortable and shameful ways of satisfying the craving. You're probably smiling at this because it seems like a reasonable way to manage binge eating, but I assure you, it is not.

It is easy to assume you have a sense of control because you're planning your binges but if you were really in control, wouldn't you be able to decide not to binge and therefore not binge? Control should be the ability to prevent a recurrence. Besides, a lot of people still eat until they feel physically sick because of the inability to stop.

You might say you take breaks like the time you had to take an urgent call or you had a visitor but be very honest, didn't you go right back when the distraction was gone? My point exactly.

Chapter 1

Why Do We Binge?

People often put on weight as a consequence of an emotional crisis in their lives. This can often be the result of a work failure, a broken friendship , a loss. However, one of the main factors why individuals start to become binge eaters is the end of a romantic relationship. I believe this is accurate, not only because of all the research on why individuals overeat but because I've encountered the same feelings and drives to eat in my own life.

Depression

Whether triggered by a chemical imbalance in the brain or a direct result of a tragic situation in one's life, it will always be detrimental to the individual's mental and therefore, physical health. This is one of the primary triggers of emotional eating. Lack of energy and loss of interest in activities that you used to enjoy will also lead to an increase in weight simply because you stop exercising as you don't see the need to get out of bed for the whole day, and pounds start to pile up. It's just a straightforward but sad reality, and it's the primary reason for emotional eating.

A second reason why depression will contribute to a rise in your weight is that your willpower will weaken and, as a consequence, your willingness not to consume unhealthy food will lose strength. The voice in your head that used to say that it's not good to eat at McDonald's every day will be replaced by the one telling you that going to McDonald's every day is the only good thing that will happen to you. The longer you'll hold this belief, the harder it will be to stop. Remaining on this route for too long, you risk getting to the point of no return and going back to a normal, healthy lifestyle will seem nearly impossible.

Loss of Command

The feeling of not being in charge of your own destiny, which is very common when a relationship ends, is also a trigger for emotional eating. We all want to be the master of our own lives and realizing that our happiness lies heavily on other people's hands can be very frustrating. Therefore, when something that we consider terrible happens, something that we can't control, we freak out. Binge eating gives you the (wrong) impression that your life is back in control.

If you're interested in losing weight and living a healthier lifestyle, click on my blog to figure out precisely how these objectives can be achieved. People are willing to take important steps when they set their minds to it. A strong degree of determination combined with the correct instruments and understanding, and the world is your oyster!

Believe it and begin living a healthy lifestyle that you owe to your buddies, your family, and most importantly, that's something you owe to yourself.

What are the Causes of Emotional Eating?.

The causes of Emotional Eating are hard to define and vary from individual to individual. However, there are some causes that often trigger overeating. Knowing what they are is a significant stage in the cycle of healing.

Here are some of the most common triggers of emotional overeating:

1. Boredom- Boredom often contributes to restlessness and the simplest way to solve it is for most individuals to consume food. The problem with eating out of boredom is that we often fail to understand how much we've consumed. It's as if our mind has lost track of what we're doing.

2. Loneliness-Often, individuals who feel lonely, particularly after a bad divorce, tend to "drown their sorrows" in meals. Some food can indeed make us feel happy but only for a very short time. This isn't terrible, but it can be harmful if we want to have a long-lasting weight loss.

3. Stress–Stress is likely the most common source of binge eating. The pressure pushes our body into a kind of inner turmoil and we look for the soothing power of food. It doesn't fix any of the issues, but we're going to eat it anyway.

4. Tiredness-Now that's interesting because fatigue isn't an emotion. Still, we often turn to food to keep us awake, especially if we have to spend some time at work or school and can't go to bed. Food can act as a transitional reservoir of energy, but it will not heal fatigue in the long run.

There are more, lesser known causes for emotional eating. After you have recognized yours, it's time to start dealing with them, one by one. It can be done. Really.

Dealing with The Factors That Leads to Emotional Eating.

When food is consumed to fulfill one's emotions instead of fulfilling one's hunger, it results in emotional eating that has adverse implications, such as the enhanced danger of heart disease, signs of anxiety and depression, and increased risk of obesity and diabetes. This research looked at the dangers of emotional eating in the hope of providing clinicians with a more substantial knowledge of how to avoid emotional eating. There is a multitude of threats deriving from emotional eating. Besides, this research explored whether one's level of fitness was correlated with emotional eating. An effort to reproduce prior connections between parenting style, one's transfers to college, and parental bonding was made using steps that permitted a more thorough assessment and the use of these factors as multi-regression predictors. Besides, gender, ethnicity estimated 27 percent of the variance seen in emotional eating and this suggest that treatment should focus on studying efficient coping techniques to reduce sensitive consumption. This research may also assist clinicians and dieticians to better understand the hazards that contribute to emotional eating.

Good and Bad Eating Habits

Children with inadequate eating habits are more likely to become overweight (or underweight). It has become a huge problem nowadays: poor dietary habits often result in overconsumption of sugar and fats and underconsumption of fiber and vitamins. Although poor eating practices can only be a component of the cause, they contribute considerably to the danger of obesity and malnutrition. This can lead to serious health issues (e.g., heart and liver illness, diabetes), particularly if these bad dietary habits are maintained through adulthood.

Bad Habits

Over-consumption of products rich in sugar, fat, and salt.

Eating unhealthy meals.

Eating when you're not hungry.

Eating small quantities (or no quantity at all) of fruit and vegetables

Eating too quickly.

Being picky eaters (to eat a restricted diet consisting of fats, carbs and sugar).

Eating while watching TV, playing video / PC games, etc.

Overeating & eating convenience.

Drinking too many sodas or sugary drinks

Skipping breakfast and dining at uneven hours.

Good Habits

Chewing your food at least 10 seconds before swallowing.

Packing a home-made lunch/breakfast for college, make sure it involves a nutritious meal (e.g., sliced fruit, pure or oat sandwiches).

Eating slowly, as it requires a few minutes for the brain to recognize that the stomach is full.

Drinking a glass of water or a bowl of soup to prevent overeating.

Scheduling time for your meal / eat on time.

Getting more fiber (e.g., whole beans and legumes).

Eating smaller servings of food.

Drinking plenty of bottled water.

Eating a range of foods per meal.

Choosing products that are steam-cooked, boiled or grilled instead of deep-fried.

Parents can be an excellent role model, practice healthy eating practices and prepare healthier products.

Avoid making a habit of dining out or ordering takeouts.

Starting to convince young people to eat healthily.

Eating together as a family as often as possible.

Avoiding treating or promising meals as a prize.

Stopping forcing your child to eat something they don't like, try to talk them into eating healthier food

Last but not least: run, exercise, play with your children, laugh and enjoy life!

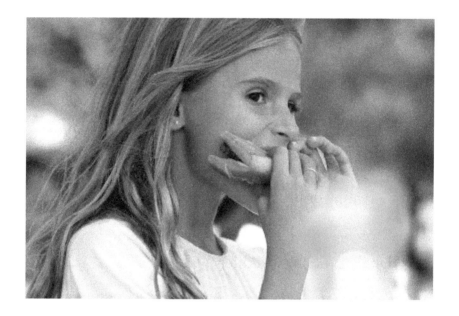

Chapter 2

Why Binging Is Bad for You

F ood can start to become scary. How much you desire it is so challenging. Why does it taste so good to eat a loaf of bread? The amount of relief that comes along when you can hold an entire gallon of ice cream and eat it directly with a spoon is like the same comfort a warm blanket can bring. Binge eating can be defined as any period that is spent eating an excess of food. People will often binge unhealthy foods at first. However, those in recovery might find that they end up binging "healthy" things like vegetables, tea, and water. It is a pattern of stuffing yourself to the point where you feel both physically and mentally ill. These periods are usually done alone, and always involve a level of shame and embarrassment.

Binging isn't enjoyable, or at least isn't the entire time. At first, there's the satisfaction of the taste, texture, and security in the amount of food you're consuming. Then, by the fourth or fifth burger, or taco, or slice of pizza, it starts to set in that you shouldn't be doing that, and that you can stop at any moment. But we keep eating, hoping to numb that logical voice in our heads.

A recorded 3 to 5% of women and 2% of men suffer from a binge eating disorder. However, many more go undiagnosed because of the stigma that surrounds eating disorders. Those who have never suffered from an eating disorder won't be the most understanding about it, either. When you have bulimia, people might recognize that you are doing something unhealthy, and this is when people start to get serious. Throwing up over and over again can mess up your body on the inside, destroying your throat and liver. Anorexia and binge eating are dangerous as well. Still, people won't always initially see these as dangerous acts, especially if you are over or under weight. Those who are underweight that binge eat don't seem like they have a problem. Some people might even look at you and make comments like, "you should gain weight," or "you are all skin and bones!" The same goes for those who are overweight and anorexic. If you go through periods of starvation as a person that's 275 pounds, people aren't going to be as concerned. Some might even encourage this behavior. Those statistics make up almost 1 out of 20 people you will meet. Yet, we still have so many confused ideologies around binge eating, overeating, anorexia, and bulimia.

Many people with binge eating disorders might develop anorexia or bulimia in response to the binge periods, or they might have had them, first which led to the binging. Either way, both are very unhealthy and can cause a person to live in shame and agony that only makes their condition worse. We do unhealthy things, and then try to do things we think are healthy to remedy them. But these are still unhealthy things. Those who suffer from anorexia and bulimia might do this because they think it is better for their bodies, as a way to respond to the overeating they put it through, first. In reality, though, it's just another unhealthy coping mechanism.

Chapter 3

Tips and Strategies to Control Your Binging

Stop Restricting Calories

If you suffer from BED, you need to stop restricting your calories. Restricting your calories was probably the reason you developed the disorder in the first place. That means giving up control over your eating behaviors and food is what you need to focus on now. Don't count calories, don't size your portions, or eat at specific times and leave out essential food groups. Forget about everything you've learned from the diet industry and start eating intuitively and listening to your body's needs!

Nature has provided us with a body that is able to give us signs that tell us when we are hungry and when not. Why not just learn to listen to it and go back to what we've practiced when we were little babies.

Babies cry when they feel hungry and want to eat, and they stop when they're full and satisfied. One day babies eat twice as much as they usually would eat, and on another day they barely eat anything. This is how biology and a healthy relationship towards food work. There's no need for us to control our body and our hunger. Nature has already provided our body with the ability to do this on its own without us needing to interrupt the natural process.

Stop Dieting

Food is not only a number, it is valuable energy and an emotional experience. Therefore, eat what you love, what serves your body and satisfies you in a pleasant way, both physically and emotionally.

Over-exercising is also a form of restricting calories which will eventually lead to the development of eating disorders and other health issues. Moderate exercise is the way for long-term health as it is the only sustainable way of moving your body. Every overdoing of exercise is not sustainable long-term and will harm your body more than it helps your health. Search for a kind of exercise that you enjoy and that you can practice long-term.

Studies have already shown that our body is not a "calorie-in-and-calorie-out machine". It is quite the opposite. That means, burning calories due to massive amounts of exercise won't make you lose weight long-term.

Therefore, find something that you love and you look forward to. No matter if that means you go on a light walk in nature, or you do some yoga in your garden or you go horse riding. It is not about the amount of exercise or the calories you burn with it. It is about regaining a healthy relationship to moving your body and feeling good in your body.

Exercise has therapeutic benefits, it should give you more power and energy. Something that adds value to your life and you benefit from. Not something you hate and "must do" in order to burn the cake you've consumed in the morning. That will only lead you back to a disordered attitude towards food, your body and exercise.

Reduce Stress

In order to stabilize eating behaviors, you'll need to address sources of stress within your life. This might not be so easy for we live in a very fast-paced world, the fastest so far. Activities are increased and a demand for productivity is highest. It might even get higher in the future.

The downside is a stressed out, habit-forming generation of unhealthy individuals. Our body seeks to be healthy and anything that threatens that would prompt the body to seek a coping mechanism. Binge eating is one method that the body uses to cope with stress. Therefore, I recommend that you eliminate stress as much as you can, and binge eating goes out of the window too.

Sleep More

The number of hours and quality of your sleep contribute a lot to your eating behaviors.

The fewer hours you sleep and if the quality is poor, the more food you'll consume to make up for your lack of energy. We often hear people encourage less sleep as a way of getting more out of life, but this is negligent. There is nothing more careless than encouraging an individual to sleep less when what they need is actually more sleep. Sleeping too little has tremendous adverse side effects which will affect your hormonal health, your brain function, your aging process, your appetite and hunger feelings and it will worsen your mental health situation long-term.

Again, it is advisable to listen to your body and get enough sleep in order to stabilize hunger and appetite.

Search for the Underlying Issue

Since every eating disorder is a mental illness, it is crucial to find the root cause of your disorder. You have to recognize that the eating disorder itself is not the main issue, it's just a symptom. The main issue is what your body is protecting you from by making you binge out on food.

You can do this by noting events that occur before you started to binge eat or that make you binge eat. Be patient about it and stay observant.

Ask yourself questions like:

What happens before I binge out on food?

How do I feel before I am about to binge and what feelings and emotions do I have during the process of binge eating?

What stresses me out in my life at the moment?

How's my family doing and how's my partner/spouse doing?

How are my relationships?

Be specific and observant and try to analyze your current life situation in order to be able to find the roots of your eating struggles.

"An eating disorder is your body's information tool that something's going on inside of you. "

Build Emotional Strength

Emotional stability and mental strength are very important when it comes to your eating behaviors and life in general. Our brain connects food with happiness and if you're emotionally dependent on the behaviors of others, you'll binge out on food as soon as those people behave in harmful ways towards you. Learn to be in love with yourself. Find happiness from within and build emotional independence.

Don't let other people and outer events control your life and how you feel about yourself. Be aware of every thought that you have because they are the roots of the emotions that you create in your body. With every thought you have, you plant the seed for a future emotion that is followed by a certain action.

If you think and focus on what other people say about you behind your back, then you plant the seed of emotions of anger, disappointment, frustration and a lack of worthiness which will eventually lead you to take certain actions such as eating food in order to compensate with these negative emotions.

Therefore, focus on yourself, your life, your health and your happiness, and not how other people try to put you down and make you feel bad about yourself.

"See your life through your own eyes and not through the eyes of others."

Practice Self-Love

Self-love and body-acceptance are crucial parts in recovering from eating disorders and it is important to emphasize them as many times as possible. Unconditionally loving your body and your personality is the real source for excellent health and happiness long-term!

In today's world we always tend to think that we are only lovable and attractive when we lose a certain amount of weight. We define ourselves through our outward appearance most times to a dangerous effect. This leads us to doing all sorts of unhealthy things just to appeal to the social construct of what beauty is. It can lead to starvation, over-exercising, and other dangerous habits.

Weight loss seems to be the tool for achieving everything in life: If we lose weight, we will be happy. If we lose weight, we will attract the partner of our life. If we lose weight, we will be successful and have the career we've always strived for. If we lose weight, we will have the best life we've always dreamed of. The list goes on.

However, the fact is, studies show that most people who lose weight are neither happier, more successful nor have a better dating life or relationships. It seems to be quite the opposite. People remain in their unsatisfied state and nothing changes for the better.

The reason for it is because of their mindset. Weight loss means losing body fat, muscle mass, and water weight. But it doesn't lead to a change in a person's mind. The mindset a person has before weight loss will remain still after they lose the weight. If a person doesn't like their body and their own personality before weight loss, they probably don't like themselves and their body after since there's only a physical change but not a mental one.

Most people tell me they are truly only able to love themselves when they lose weight but that is a wrong expectation because it is not that they start loving themselves more after weight loss.

No, it is that they start loving their "lighter" body and how they look on the outside but that is not the same as "truly and deeply loving themselves." Self-love is not the same as "body-love" to be fair. Self-love includes body-love but body-love doesn't necessarily include self-love. Self-love is beyond more than only loving your body and outward appearance, in fact, it is independent from your outward appearance and your weight.

It is loving yourself in every aspect of your life, accepting yourself as who you are and as a whole human being. Allowing your body to have some stretch marks and some cellulite on the thighs, allowing yourself not to be motivated and perfect every single day and stop seeing yourself as an incomplete being.

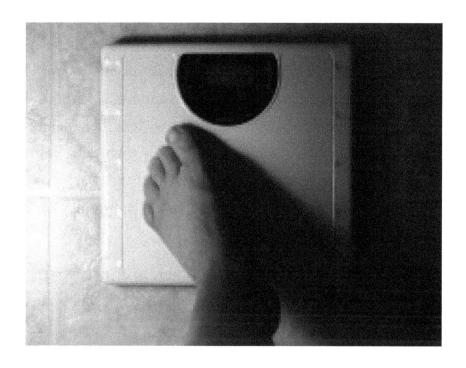

Chapter 4

The Importance of Meditation & Self-Awareness

We often overeat because we feel anxious, worried, frustrated, or think negatively about ourselves or situations. When this happens, we can turn to mindful meditation so we can change our mind-set and start to focus on believing the positive things about ourselves and what we can achieve.

If you've done any form of meditation, you will be able to achieve mindful meditation as it's similar to other forms of meditation. When we meditate, we work on cleaning out the clutter in our minds, so we no longer have cloudy thoughts but clear thoughts. Cloudy thoughts are often the thoughts that bring in the negative light we see around ourselves as it clouds our vision. When we have clear thoughts, that negativity is gone, and we can fully focus on the positive light we have around us.

The first step to meditation is you want to find a quiet spot you can focus. You want to make sure this spot is free from any interruptions, which I understand in the life of a millennial can be hard to find. If you're struggling because of a family and young children, try to find time to practice your mindful meditation before you go to be or get up early in the morning before everyone else wakes up. It's important that you're able to take time to yourself to meditate so you don't lose focus.

Once you have found your quiet spot where you won't become interrupted, you can lie down or sit down in a comfortable position. You might find it comfortable to sit with your legs crossed, similar to the states of Buddha. You might find it more comfortable to sit with your feet flat on the floor or lie down on your back. No matter what position you find comfortable, you want to make sure you're comfortable so you can focus on what you need to focus on during meditation.

Next, you want to close your eyes and do your best to clear your mind of any cloudy thoughts. You need to have your mind as clear as possible before we start focusing on the breathing exercises in the next step. I understand this won't be easy at first, and from time to time, you will let your mind drift as you start thinking of something. This happens to everyone when they start to meditate. The key here is to be kind to yourself. Don't be hard on yourself because you let your mind wander. Just focus on getting rid of those negative thoughts again and then continue your meditation.

Once your mind is clear, you can start to focus on your regular breathing. During this time, you will only focus on your breathing. With your eyes closed, put one hand on your stomach and the other hand on your chest and breathe normally. As you breathe, notice the movements of your stomach and your chest. You can also feel the clothes on your skin as they move with every breath you take.

Next, you want to take deep breaths. Keep your hands in place with one resting on your chest and the other resting on your stomach as you take a deep breath in and out? Breathe in slowly and then release your breath slowly. As you do this, focus on your hands. Notice how the hand on your stomach rises up whenever you take a deep breath in and then falls with your stomach when you exhale. Continue to focus on your breathing in meditation for about ten minutes. Remember, if you catch your mind wandering, simply focus on clearing your thoughts.

Chapter 5

The Importance of Diet & Exercise

D id you know that you should consider exercises that may enable you to oppose desires to eat or upchuck? These will be required for the hour or so when the inclinations are at their generally extraordinary. Individuals' selections of exercises vary, however here are some run of the mill ones:

- Taking an energetic walk or bike ride
- Calling or visiting companions or relatives
- Working out
- Messaging
- Going on Facebook
- Perusing the Web
- Playing a computer game
- Scrubbing down or shower
- Watching a drawing in motion picture or a most loved TV program

The objective is that you make a rundown of exercises that suits you actually. As a rule, every movement needs to have three properties:

1. It is dynamic (i.e., it includes accomplishing something) instead of uninvolved, (for example, watching whatever happens to be on TV).

2. It is pleasant (i.e., it doesn't feel like a task).

3. It is sensible (i.e., it is something that you are probably going to do).

Here is another valuable tip.

Experience your music accumulation and distinguish bits of music that you appreciate and mind-set improving. You may well find that music is great at changing your outlook and consequently at helping you manage desires to eat or upchuck.

Keep such music close by, prepared for use at troublesome occasions. In reality, you may get a kick out of the chance to make a particular playlist for this reason.

When you have built your rundown of exercises, record them on a card or keep an e-note of them some place convenient. Your rundown should be promptly gotten to at whatever point you have inclinations to eat or upchuck.

You likewise need to get master at distinguishing these inclinations. It is critical to spot them early when they are simpler to manage.

Along these lines, when you identify an inclination of this sort, note it down in segment 6 of your observing record and get out your rundown of elective exercises.

Substituting Elective Exercises: What to Do

You have to work on taking part in elective exercises when you experience inclinations to eat or upchuck. Evaluate your advancement at every one of your audit sessions. Likewise, make sure to finish your rundown sheet every week. Order as a "change day" any day on which you checked precisely; you clung to week by week gauging; you put forth a valiant effort to adhere to your arranged example of ordinary eating, as portrayed in Stage 2, regardless of whether you likewise gorged; and you utilized your rundown of elective exercises to manage desires to eat or upchuck.

Survey Sessions

At each survey session you should think about your checking records and synopsis sheet (finished week by week) and ask yourself the four inquiries underneath, notwithstanding those identifying with Stages 1 and 2.

1. Have I contrived a rundown of elective exercises? You ought to have made a rundown and be conveying it with you. On the off chance that you are to mediate when you have to, you will require this rundown nearby. The rundown may well require change based on understanding: a few exercises may work; others may not.

2. Am I recording desires to eat or upchuck? You ought to record these desires in segment 6 of your observing records. In the event that you are to intercede effectively, you should record these desires at the time that you experience them as opposed to sometime a while later.

Glance through the checking records that you have finished since beginning Stage 3. Have there been inclinations to eat or upchuck? Did you record them when they happened? On the off chance that you have been eating now and again other than your arranged dinners and bites, this proposes you have had such desires.

3. Am I utilizing my rundown of elective exercises when required? On the off chance that you have had a desire to eat between your dinners and snacks, or to upchuck, have you utilized your rundown of exercises?

4. Could my utilization of elective exercises be improved? In the event that you have endeavored to intercede, how could it go? Did you mediate early enough? Did you take part in at least one

of the exercises on your rundown? Which exercises worked, and which didn't? Have you adjusted your rundown as needs be?

It is ideal to have a survey session like this at any rate a few times per week.

At this phase in the program, almost certainly, you will infer that there has been practically no adjustment in your weight. In any case, we have to think about two potential outcomes.

1. Your weight has fallen reliably since beginning the program, and you are presently underweight. If so, you should see your doctor, clarify what you have been doing, and get counsel. The program may not be appropriate for you. It is conceivable that you are eating excessively small during your suppers and tidbits. This is a potential issue since it will constrain your capacity to stop overeating.

2. Your weight has risen reliably while following the program. On the off chance that this applies, you have to check two things. The first is whether you are currently "overweight," restoratively. If so, you should examine this issue with your doctor. On the off chance that you choose to do this, you ought to clarify that you are following a logically tried program that is intended to enable you to recover command over your eating. It's anything but a get-healthy plan. As we noted before, you will be in a vastly improved situation to

control your weight once you have authority over your eating.

The subsequent issue to consider is whether you were to some degree underweight when you began the program. Assuming this is the case, it isn't improbable that your weight is presently expanding to an increasingly solid level. This is something worth being thankful for, despite the fact that you might think that it's hard to acknowledge.

What you should not do is go on an exacting eating routine since this would probably fix any advancement you have made up until this point.

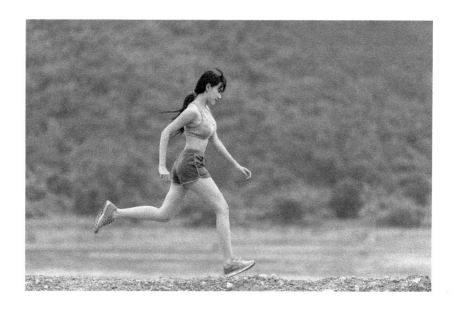

Chapter 6

Should I Seek Professional Help? Nutritionists, Psychotherapy and Medication

There are some types of medication that can be used in treating binge eating. Remember though that medicines are not to be relied on as the sole means of treating the problem. It can help in relieving some of the symptoms and effects of the disorder, but it can never be used in treating the cause and reversing it.

With that in mind, here are some of the common medications prescribed for treating Binge Eating Disorders:

Appetite Suppressants

Appetite suppressants are some of the most common drugs used for treating binge eating. One of the reasons this drug is used is because most patients who suffer from BED would also like to lose weight.

The psychotherapy that they are undergoing might do nothing for you when it comes to weight reduction. Appetite suppressants on the other hand promise some weight loss. Though you need to eat less as well.

This type of drug was first used for treating BED during the 90s. The problem was that one of the first appetite suppressing drugs used for this purpose was found to have some very harmful effects on the body. The risks included a high rate of cardiovascular diseases and other unwanted side effect.

Learning proper portion control and choosing healthier foods is the best approach and even if you use appetite suppressants, you'll still need to choose your foods wisely.

Current Drugs

Today the most common drug used for treating binge eating by suppressing appetite and causing weight loss is Orlistat. This drug affects the ability of the body to absorb fat which in turn prevents the body from gaining weight.

In reality it really is not an appetite suppressant. Orlistat works by binding to the molecules of the fat in the food and preventing it from being broken down by the stomach into components that are easier to absorb.

There are other drugs currently being considered for use in controlling the appetite of those who are suffering from binge eating disorder. There are problems though with the side effects caused by these drugs. Some side effects include impairment of the patient's cognitive ability. Another side effect that has been reported is that of tingling and numbness of the skin. This is not to say that Orilstat doesn't have unpleasant side effects, and if you are thinking about using it, you'll want to discuss this carefully with your doctor.

Topamax

Topiramate which is another name for Topamax is a drug that was originally intended for treating seizures. Some studies have suggested that it can help curb binge eating and that it could help jump start or increase weight loss.

Certain studies indicate that people suffering from Binge Eating Disorder might benefit from taking Topamax. While this use of the drug is not an officially approved or recommended use of the drug it does hold a great amount of promise for those who are suffering from this form of behavioral problem.

History of Topamax

Topamax was created for treating epilepsy and seizures. The drug was created in the late 1970s. The effect of the drug was meant to stop the convulsions of those who have epilepsy.

Aside from the treatment of epilepsy the drug has also been used for other types of diseases. It has been used to treat bipolar disease and to counteract the weight gain in other diseases. Its use for treating bipolar disease has stopped since it has been shown to offer too few benefits for that problem.

Other Uses

The drug has been used to treat other problems as well. It has been used for treating migraine and severe headache. This use is due to the effect the drug has on blood vessels in the brain. It helps to widen them. Another reason why it is effective as a migraine treatment is because it has very few side effects.

It has been used for fighting the effects of alcoholism and other behavioral problems. There are other diseases and health problems for which this drug is being used but the one that we are most interested in is its effect on those who have Binge Eating Disorder.

Topamax for Binge Eating Disorder

Although the use of Topamax for BED is not really recommended by experts there are some very positive reviews on its effects. Studies conducted indicate that people who are suffering from BED were able to control their eating and their appetite by taking Topamax.

Those who used the drug had less attacks of binge eating, lost weight and even experienced a great amount of loss in their BMI. People who used the drug were able to lose as much as a pound per week over a 14-week period. Though this is not an officially approved use of the drug it does show a lot of promise for those having to cope with binge eating.

Topamax Usage

There are some reminders about Topamax usage I'd like to share:

1.   Anyone taking the drug should stay away from activities that require a certain level of mental alertness. The drug might impair abilities in that area.

2.   The use of the drug can affect the way that the body regulates heat so if taking Topamax, you should refrain from activities that can increase body heat.

3.   Topamax can decrease the effectiveness of certain contraceptives.

4.   The sudden discontinuation of the use of the drug should be discouraged because it might cause a sudden increase in the number of seizures.

There are cases of overdose of this drug, but they are very rare. The more serious cases of problems with the drug were instances where it had been used in conjunction with other medications. Overdose can cause several symptoms and they might include depression, blurred vision, problems with speech and thinking.

Before taking Topamax or any drug for that matter, in order to treat your Binge Eating Disorder make sure that you consult your doctor first so that s/he can give you the best advice.

Under No Circumstances Should You Take Any Drug without Your Doctor's Permission and Consent.

Antidepressants

Another type of drug that is often used for treating BED are antidepressants. Recent research has proven this effect of the drug although long term studies are lacking.

There were seven studies conducted where the results showed promise that antidepressants might be able to help those who are suffering from BED. Over 40% of people who suffered from BED and took part in the studies had positive results after taking in anti-depressants.

The Use of Anti-Depressants

Antidepressants are used for alleviating the mood of those who suffer from depression and other forms of mood disorders. This kind of drug can have an alleviating effect on those with mood problems, but they do not have the same effect on normal people. Usually this kind of drug has delayed effect of about 3 to 6 weeks and its use is usually prescribed for a period that lasts for months to years.

Side Effects

There are certain side effects that come with the use of antidepressants. These side effects include nausea, dry mouth, dizziness, constipation and sleepiness. There are other types of side effects as well depending on the drug taken.

Use of Antidepressants in Fighting BED

The use of antidepressants when it comes to fighting the effects of Binge Eating Disorder seems promising, but you need to keep in mind that it has not been officially recommended for that use. There are also some risks involved including relapse if you discontinue using the drug.

Self-Prescriptions

The medications listed here have shown indications that they can be beneficial when it comes to treating Binge Eating Disorder. However, you should never use them on your own. Even if these are not officially prescribed as medications for binge eating you should still consult a doctor before you take any of these medications.

As you have seen, some of the drugs have some adverse side effects. This information I have researched on these drugs is offered to you so you can talk to your doctor about your options in your specific case. You always seek the guidance of a physician before you use any drug.

Chapter 7

Health Problems Caused by Binge Eating

H ere are some major health problems that you should be searching for. Know what you can do about each of them.

Weight Gain and Obesity Weight Gain is normal when you eat binge. Two-thirds of those with this condition are overweight. You put on extra pounds by eating a lot of food in a short period of time and not running off your calories from exercise.

A lot of people who overweight still feel bad for their weight.

It leads to low self-esteem, which can lead to more overeating. Overweight or obese may also increase your chances of having long-term health issues, such as:

- Breathing that slows several times during the night (sleep apnea)

- Diabetes

- Heart disease

- High blood pressure

- Type 2 diabetes

- Arthritis

The clothing will start to feel tight. The figures on the size of your bathroom are going up. A doctor will check how much body fat you have by measuring:

• Weight to height ratio (Body Mass Index, or BMI)

• Abdominal size using a tape measure placed above the waist and around the center of the body (around the waist)

Tests are performed to check blood pressure, blood sugar, and cholesterol levels—all of which may be impaired by weight gain.

Treatment for binge eating coincides by working out why you're overeating.

This is what you need to do before you try to lose weight. The doctor and the psychiatrist will help you get going. First, plan to talk to a dietitian and come up with a diet and exercise schedule that you can stick with. Tell them for advice on how to live at a healthy weight.

Heart Disease getting overweight makes it harder for your heart to pump oxygen to your lungs and body. Having a lot of weight, particularly around the belly, increases your risk of high blood pressure, high cholesterol, and high blood sugar. All of these things raise the risk of heart attack and stroke.

Sometimes there are no signs of heart disease, so it's hard to know that you have it. Here are a few warning signs:

• Pain in the cheat area

• Fainting or Dizziness

• Rapid pulse

• Shortness of breath

• Sweating: Eat a healthy diet and exercise regularly.

Such factors protect your heart from injury and raising the risk of heart disease. Ask your doctor or dietitian for ways to eat healthy and workout safely. You may also need drugs to reduce the blood pressure, cholesterol, and blood sugar.

Type 2 Diabetes Studies show that people who eat binge are more likely to have type 2 diabetes. Diabetes can be a life-long illness that requires ongoing treatment. If you have this disorder, binge eating will make your blood sugar more difficult to control.

• Blurry vision

• Constant nausea or fatigue

• Fatigue

• Need to pee more often than normal

• Numbness or tingling in your hands and feet Check your blood sugar as often as the doctor suggests. If you do not know how to do this at home, contact your doctor who will let you know. Always ask her to tell you what the target of your blood sugar is.

Here are some ways to regulate your blood sugar: • Eat more fruit, vegetables and whole grains. Have a little less fat and sugar.

• Drink water instead of fruit or coffee.

• Train most days of the week.

• Taking any medications for diabetes that your doctor recommends.

Depression and Other Mood Disorders Depression and anxiety are more common in people with binge eating disorders. A lot of people who eat binge do that kind of stuff to improve their mood. This can lead to feelings of remorse that make you drink more.

Overeating when you're not hungry may be an indication that you're trying to dull your emotions. They may also feel:

• Depressed or powerless

• Angry

• Like you don't have much value in things that you once enjoyed

• Lonely or lonely all the time

• Tired, feeling like you don't have any strength

Many therapies for binge eating disorder may avoid both the excessive eating and the lonely attitude that sometimes goes with it. These include:

• Cognitive behavioral therapy (CBT). This will make you feel better about yourself, prevents the negative feelings that cause you to binge

• Antidepressants, which can boost your wellbeing and also help to combat binge when you need to go to Hospital Rarely, binge eating disorders can be severe enough to treat you in a hospital.

Here are some signs that you need professional help right away:

• You gained or lost weight in a concise time.

• You were talking about hurting yourself.

• You can't change the way you live, even with the aid of doctors, relatives, and friends.

• You're either depressed or anxious.

• You used drugs or alcohol to deal with your feelings.

Ways to reset after a Binge

1. Don't beat yourself up, man.

Anyone who's been there knows the feeling. The worst is the result of a binge.

"Emotionally and mentally, you've just ruined yourself," "People that drink, it's very hasty, thrilling... It's like someone hunting for a drug. Nutrition is a drug to binge men. So the frustration and worry to find out how you're going to get what you want, to do it and get it done before you're exposed... You're done. "That's just the beginning.

Once you're done with your binge, all the negative emotions tend to pile up.

"There's a lot of shame, a lot of hopelessness, they also feel a lot more frustration towards themselves," "you just get that overwhelming feeling,' I just ruined it,'" "Perhaps the first thing you should know after a relapse is — it occurs.

"One of the stuff I still tell people is... you're going to gorge," that's how we create endurance, that's how we develop the ability to make course correct. It's how we know how to live in rehab. "She's a well-recovered binge eater.

"Recovery's never going to drink again. It's about' less and less repeated and less and less earnest, and we're much easier able to get out of the loop, understand what's happened, and satisfy those needs in other ways.

"That's what healing is — never to drink again." In other words, after one happens, go easy on yourself.

"I still say you're going to have to get over the shame. You can't change it," "It's not like you've got the super-powers and you can push the clock back an hour. It's over," "It's straightforward to beat yourself. But nothing good ever comes out of self-torture. "Rather, take the time to take care of yourself, to" befriend "your body, as Pershing puts it. Realize that this is your home, not an advertisement that you're showing the world.

"Imagine saying to yourself,' my body is just as worthy of love and respect now as it was before the binge,'" "What do I need right now to take care of my body at this moment?

2. Figure out what's gone wrong.

Post-binge is the time for a bit of sleuthing. What could have set the binge off? Is it hunger? (Bingers sometimes gorge at a binge, setting off a chain that is sometimes hard to break.) Sadness? A bad experience with someone, huh?

"You need to be really honest about why you haven't done this for three weeks, and why did it happen again," she said, "What's going on in my relationship? Am I just tired, huh? Am I always sick of that? See it as a source of information.' Whatever it is, define it and recognize it. That might support you next time around.

"Recognizing what's going on with the relapse and then taking a few steps forward can actually help you avoid it becoming a weekly occurrence, for example," is really important to get back on track as soon as possible.

3. Please stick to your timetable.

Kearney-Cooke has a simple routine for the binge. It's time to brush your teeth. It means an end to the addiction and a return to a fresh approach to wellness.

"The way a lot of bingers sound is,' Damn, I've lost it. I'm going to let it go,' I want them to start by saying,' Yeah, I've been binged.

So, for the next 24 hours, I'm going to get back to healthy eating right away.' "That doesn't mean eating or not eating— what psychologists call" restricting"— trying to make up for the binge. That often translates to more of a spree.

The goal is to get back to your regular schedule, including your workout. Hitting the gym can help you deal with the stress of a binge, and it can help the attitude, too.

4. Get out of here and go.

Most binges are kept in a bar or in front of family or friends.

"It's really a disease of loneliness," to leave the binge behind or not to have another one, also helps to get out of the house and away from the kitchen and take some time doing something you like to do. You're walking your horse. Off to a game, man. Having a college.

"As soon as a person understands that food is not the only thing you can use to take away depression, suffering, rage, sadness — that there are so many other really great things to do," "As soon as they realize that and choose another hobby or several activities, it becomes easier and easier for a person to remove himself from the food."

5. Get out of there for help.

Find family, friends, and experts who can help you out. Several people and organizations, including online groups of people battling binge eating, are there for you. About 1% to 5% of Americans have binge eating disorders. Some of the more than 30 million Americans will have an eating disorder in their lifetime.

You're not alone here.

"It's not something people usually think about. There's a lot of shame about it. And it's also embarrassing for them to see what's going on; they avoid thinking about it and learning about it, "It certainly takes a lot of courage and bravery to confront it. But if you admit it, there's a lot of proper treatment out there. And it can actually improve the quality of your life.

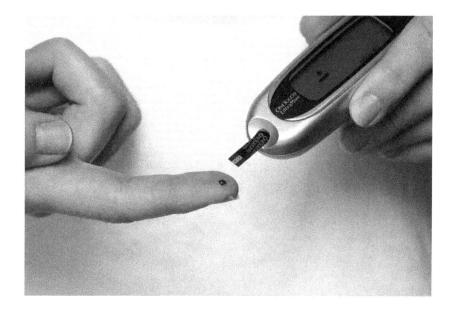

Chapter 8

How to Lose Weight

Let's dive into the four-step process of weight loss to remove some of the confusion around losing weight.

The central concept that allows people to be sustainable with their weight loss is the idea of autonomy. That is, you have control over your decisions on how to lose weight.

The actual process of losing weight is biological. How you go about it involves a lot of options and choices available to you. Let's examine the four-step process, which gives you a lot of flexibility. The four-step process involves certain principles that have to be present. How you go about implementing them is up to you. Now the first one - create a calorie deficit. You cannot lose weight unless you are in a calorie deficit. The alternatives to a calorie deficit are either a calorie surplus, in which case you are consuming more than you are expending or calorie maintenance, in which case both calorie expenditure and calorie intake are equal, in which case you will not lose or gain weight.

Typically, a person wants to lose weight, and so they dust off their running shoes, and they go running, or they go to the gym four or five times a week when previously they didn't go at all. What happens is they do it to try to increase their energy expenditure, following the idea that if you exercise more, you lose weight.

Two things will happen, though; one is your hunger will increase because you are placing new demands on the body. Also, and this is just anecdotal, but I find a familiar pattern, is what tends to happen is compromise appears in mind. It's "I have done this," "I deserve this." "I've exercised three times this week, and I deserve a little treat." That treat tends to be the thing that you've taken away, and what tends to happen is that treat causes you to overeat. We also tend to overestimate the amount of energy expended with exercise; we over anticipate it.

Increasing your NEAT, everyday movement is what you want to do every day. That includes things like walking more, taking the stairs instead of the lift, gardening, when you are making a cup of tea or coffee do five squats, and get up from your desk a lot more.

One of the common traits that occur for naturally lean people is they fidget a lot. Fidgeting is a biological act, I can't say to you start to fidget; it's not going to happen. The next best thing is moving a lot more in everyday life.

The fourth one is to mitigate SODIT moments. SODIT is an acronym for all the things that occur that are most likely to cause you to stray from your eating plan. SODIT stands for stress, overwhelmed, distraction, internal dialogue, and tiredness.

When you are stressed, you are more likely to say, "SODIT, I'm going to eat this; I'm going to have a takeaway pizza."

When you are in overwhelm, anxious, and on the go, again it's, "Oh, I'll get this quickly, I'll get this quickly. I'm on the move. I need to eat something."

Distraction are those things where you are like, "Oh, I got that holiday at the weekend. I got that event in two weeks. Oh, I've got this meeting that lasted longer than I expected." These are distraction moments that create a decision point of, "Well, I haven't had anything, so I'm going to get something from the vendor machine," all the things that mean that you stray away from your proposed plan of how you were going to eat.

Internal dialogue is things like "Oh, I've always failed. Ugh, this is so boring. Why do I bother?" All of those internal dialogues are going to influence your decision on what to eat.

The final one is the tiredness. Hormonal tiredness can do things such as increasing the level of Ghrelin which is an appetite enhancer, you might end up getting brain fog where you are not thinking as clearly as you could be, and you end up grabbing anything that you can.

All these moments can happen regularly, but we want to mitigate them, so we always feel like we are on the road to success; we still feel in control.

That's the four-step process. We want to make it as simple as possible. As you can see, there's a lot of places where you can have your input. I haven't told you, "Oh, you must follow this 28-day plan." All of those areas can be altered based on your lifestyle.

Chapter 9

Creating a Healthy Food Plan for Long-Term Results

H ere are just some of the most efficient ways you can create a food plan for your own health, and actually stick to it:

1. Do not try to avoid shopping. Most people suffering from BED try their very best to avoid going to the supermarket for fear of triggering the binge. Some even go as far as not keeping their kitchen pantries adequately stocked. As a result, they may end up not eating enough—and because they're too hungry, they might fall into the trap of bingeing on unhealthy processed food instead.

This is why it's important to plan your meals—and your ingredients—in advance. Of course, you shouldn't plan a rigid schedule that's set in stone. You might be forced to adhere to it on an extremely strict basis—this will only lead to more risks of getting stuck inside the BED cycle. You should, however, establish a structure around eating. This structure helps dial down the fear around food and grocery shopping.

2. Work with your dietician. That said, you need to come up with about five ideas on balanced breakfasts, lunches, dinners, and snacks—yes, you need to plan for snacks too so that you don't binge on junk food. These options will assist you in making good choices during mealtime. Take about ten minutes every week to plan the meals that will get you through the whole seven days, and make a list of ingredients and recipes for them. Keep in mind that most of the healthier meal alternatives out there are more perishable than the processed ones, so take note of those expiration dates as well.

Just in case you don't have the time to cook your own meals, you can head on over to the prepared section of your local market and look for balanced meals you can easily put together there.

3. Make room for spontaneous events. Just because you have already planned for the whole week doesn't mean you can't have a nice dinner out with a friend. On any given day, just make sure that when you come home from a long and tiring day, you won't find yourself in the position of not knowing what you should prepare for your dinner.

4. Try to make meals out of the different food groups out there. Go for vegetables, proteins, starches, and even fat, as long as everything is balanced. Even some fat can help make your meal taste better. Remember that you should never completely forbid a certain type of food in your house or you will only want

it more. It's okay to keep your own trigger foods at bay, but everything should still always be in moderation. If you're unsure about what to include in your meal, divide your whole plate into thirds. For instance, aim for a third of starch, a third of protein, and a third of fruits and veggies.

5. When in doubt, jot them down. While you're recovering from BED, you might have a hard time trying to figure out when you're emotionally hungry and when you're actually hungry. To keep your head clear, jot down how you feel along with what you are eating. This way, you can properly determine the times when your body is emotionally hungry or physically hungry.

6. Eat every three to four hours. This way, you are helping to boost your body's ability to use your food and break them down. This kind of meal spacing also trains your body to identify better if it is still full or really hungry. Do not plan for six small meals, because when you do get a regular sized meal later on, you might feel guilty about it. Instead, go for three big meals spaced accordingly, with the snacks in between.

Chapter 10

The Emotional Effect of Overeating

O vereating is often called emotional eating because we're more likely to overeat and binge eat over emotional reasons. Along with this, we often establish other emotions when we overeat as we start to feel ashamed or angry that we "let ourselves go" and had another binge eating episode. The emotional effects tend to be the same general emotions for the majority of people who suffer from binge eating. But, because we're all individuals, other emotional effects can pop up in a person that doesn't pop up in the next person. No matter what your emotions are after a binge eating episode, they contribute to the cycle which can make you continue to binge eat.

One of the biggest accomplishments when you work on overcoming your binge eating is breaking the cycle. Without breaking the cycle, none of the other steps you're accomplishing would be possible as a cycle tends to keep us going around and around within it. Cycles usually have a deep grip within people that are hard to escape. I feel it's important for you to understand how vicious the cycle is because once you do escape that cycle, you should be proud of yourself. You should note this accomplishment because cycles are very hard to break, especially after you've lived within them for a long period of time.

Nausea

Whenever we overeat, we tend to feel a little nauseous as this is our body's way of telling us we ate too much, too fast, and it's working hard in order to process the calories. Because we ate too much, it would take longer for our body's organ to work through all the food.

Nauseous is never a good feeling for anyone. Even if we don't have any other symptoms, like you would if you had a stomach bug or flu, it tends to make us feel more miserable than before. Some people become sluggish, and due to not feeling well, they go to lie down. These effects of nausea contribute to people's vicious cycle who just had a binge eating episode. Because they're aware that they ate too much and made themselves not feel well, they tend to have other emotional effects of eating too much.

Guilt

Guilt is one of the most common emotional effects of binge eating. When we start to feel guilt over our actions, we allow our negative emotions to take over our thoughts. We start to feel the way these negative emotions tell us we feel. For example, we start to feel bad about what we just did to ourselves and wonder how we could be so stupid to be able to let this happen again. We start to tell ourselves that we should know better and wonder why we didn't learn from the last time.

When you start to feel guilty about your emotional eating, you start to put yourself down. You start to tell yourself that you knew better. You're stupid for falling for that trap again. You start to emotionally beat yourself up because of the guilt you're feeling. This causes you to have low self-esteem, which holds you in this vicious cycle of binge eating as you feel that you won't ever overcome it because you're not good enough.

Humiliation and Embarrassment

Embarrassment, humiliation, and shame are other emotional side effects that tend to keep you in the cycle of binge eating. These feelings are similar to guilt for they give us low self-esteem because of the negative emotions we feel and the way we see our bodies. When you start to become embarrassed over your binge eating episode, you start to become ashamed of what you did to your body. In return, you start to become ashamed of your body and the way you believe other people see your body. You start to view yourself as obese, ugly, and feel that people laugh at you because of your size.

It's a proven fact that binge eating causes us to gain weight, and if you're a binge eater, you already know this, and you've already seen it. It's these body images that not only keep us in the cycle but can lead others into developing different eating disorders, such as bulimia and anorexia. Instead of working toward losing weight a healthy way, we often keep ourselves in this cycle due to the emotional effects of binge eating.

Another way people become embarrassed about themselves is when they realized they have an eating disorder. They feel ashamed because, as millennials, we feel we should know better. How many of us went to school and learned about eating disorders? Because of this, we feel that we should have known better and not fallen into the trap, or we should have known better to be able to stop our overeating sooner so it didn't become a problem.

Depression

Depression is another common emotional effect to recurring binge eating episodes that can lead into much bigger, sometimes life-threatening, and problems. Before I get any further into depression and binge eating, I want to tell you that if you feel so depressed that you've considered harming yourself, others, or taking your own life, please seek help immediately. I realize that this is a very sensitive issue and touchy subject for many people, but I want you to know that you are loved by so many people. You're loved by your parents, your friends, your coworkers, other family members, and people in your community and college classrooms. Your life is a precious gift, and you have so many amazing gifts that you can share with those around you. If you're not sure where to start, you can call any suicide hotline as there are many that remain open twenty-four hours a day, seven days a week, 365 days a year. You can also go into the emergency room, and a doctor will help you with the next steps. If you're a college student, your counselor's office is a great place to start. I also want you to know that you're not alone, and you don't have to fight the battle alone. Call a friend or family member as they will find ways to help you too.

Depression starts to occur as an emotional effect of binge eating due to the negative way we talk to ourselves. The more and more negative statements we feed to our self-esteem, the more likely we are to become depressed. When we start to talk down to ourselves, we start to believe ourselves, and we start to believe other people feel the same way about us. Because we aren't lifting ourselves up in positive ways, we're not going to feel positive about ourselves.

There is a difference between depression and sadness. Sadness usually only lasts for a few hours to a couple days, whereas, depression can last longer because it's a stronger emotion. There's also a difference between clinical depression, which we need treatment to overcome, and depression that lasts for a short period of time. Without spending too much more time on this effect of binge eating, I just want to take a few moments to give you some of the major symptoms of depression. It's very important to get help for depression as soon as you notice you hold some of these symptoms as just with any other disorder, such as binge eating. It continues to get worse, and before you know it, it's controlling your life instead of your controlling your emotions in your life.

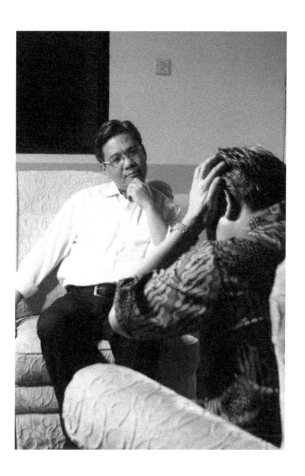

Chapter 11

Effective Ways to Curb Binge Eating

1. Get the right kind of help

Getting help for binge eating disorder will eventually involve talking to a doctor or healthcare provider. You need to be diagnosed with BED formally, and your health insurance plans (if any) may be able to help you once you have a diagnosis. Remember, binge eating disorder is now considered a formal mental health condition with a psychological component.

Everyone is different, but BED normally requires you to get a psychological evaluation. You'll probably have to answer a lot of questions about your eating habits. If necessary, you may also get follow-up tests to see whether or not BED has had a negative impact on your body. Tests will look for signs of bodily stress, such as high blood pressure, diabetes, problems with sleep, and high cholesterol.

Common tests include urine and blood tests, physical check-up, and even an appointment with a sleep expert. Once a diagnosis is confirmed, you can start treatment with the goal of finding root causes of binge eating, and ending behavior that contributes to binge eating.

You may end up having therapy in either a group or individual setting. Common therapies for people with BED are dialectical behavior therapy. The goal of this kind of therapy is to help you learn skills in order to deal with stress, emotions, and learn how to relate well to others.

Cognitive behavioral therapy (CBT) can help you learn to control better the things that trigger stress or binge eating. It can also help you make better sense of your triggers so you gain control and reclaim your life.

Interpersonal psychotherapy can help you relate to others better. If unhealthy communication with other people triggers you to binge eat, then this therapy can help you communicate with and relate to others in ways that don't leave you feeling drained.

Some doctors may also offer medication and weight-loss programs that can help you deal with binge eating. Remember, each plan will be customized depending on your needs.

2. Stop dieting

What is meant here is to stop fad dieting. People today have the tendency to employ weight-loss methods that leave out important food groups. As such, the best thing to do is to stop following diets promoted by magazines, cultural trends, and even celebrities.

Some fad diets force you to cut out entire foods that were once common to you. Although part of BED recovery involves changing how you eat, studies show that restrictive diets actually contribute to binge eating because they make the prohibited food items seem irresistible.

Many fad diets are also designed to make you lose weight fast. Food extremes are never healthy. Instead, make slow changes to your diet by adding nutritious meals that include all basic food groups. Whole grains, fresh fruit and vegetables, fiber, and protein, are all necessary parts of a healthy diet. Your doctor and other professional caregivers can help you with this if needed. Slow but steady!

For some people, it might be best not to try any dieting until they've spoken to a

Healthcare provider that can supervise their current lifestyle changes.

3. Stop skipping meals

One common way for people to feed into their binge eating disorder is to skip meals. The guilt of binge eating may make you think that skipping meals sounds sensible. However, it's best to have set meal times instead.

Fasting can actually make you more vulnerable to temptations, cause you to crave comfort foods, and contribute to binge eating even more as your physical and emotional hunger levels collide.

4. Understand how your brain is tricking you

Unlike an addiction to a substance, stopping binge eating at its tracks is different because it means you'd have to quit food. That's impossible!

As such, make sure you recognize how your brain is tricking you into wanting to find comfort in food as you go through something hard. Once you become aware of the things that are making you want to eat more, you'll be better equipped to ask yourself why you're actually eating.

This is going to take some practice, and it will most likely involve learning skills from your doctor or therapist. Remember that by identifying the things that make you seek comfort in food, you're unlearning mindless eating. Actually thinking about what you eat and when is key to making slow changes that will eventually train you to gain control of your life, emotions, and binge eating habits.

5. Hack restaurant menus

One obstacle to ending the negative cycle of binge eating is that food is unavoidable. You'll end up at a restaurant at many points in your recovery. You may be there because of a work-mandated, possibly mandatory event. A partner, friend, or family member may take you there as a treat, or they may be asking you to join them for a special occasion.

Food isn't the enemy. In binge eating, it's our attitudes, our reward center, and even the psychology of restaurant menus that can wreak havoc on our recovery. What's one to do?

Stay informed! Remember what we learned about restaurant menus. Many of them use specific color palettes to make us hungry, such as red and yellow, because research shows that this works.

Remember to stick to items to your left, if you can. Really think about your order so that you make a decision out of hunger instead of restaurant psychology. But remember that if you deprive yourself of everything you crave, you'll make your own recovery more difficult. As such, don't be too hard on yourself when you go to a restaurant.

But also, remember that you can control certain things. You can also decide to choose a venue with healthy options, and maybe being in a place that makes it easy for you to be comfortable will help you avoid overeating.

6. Find a support network

Asking for help can be difficult, and coming clean about an eating disorder such as binge eating may be hard. Not everyone is sensitive about overeating, and people tend to be more familiar with disorders such as anorexia and bulimia.

However, a 2014 analysis of studies on binge eating disorders shows that including a social network in treatment could have many benefits in people who deal with BED. This may include relying on support from friends, colleagues, members of a faith community, neighbors, family members, and intimate partners.

It's hard for people to help you tackle an unhealthy relationship with something as ubiquitous and necessary as food if they don't understand it. Including a select group of people from your social network in your recovery can have many benefits for both you, and your relationship with those you include in your journey.

7. Drink water

Many diet blogs and health experts often tell you to drink water because it can help you lose weight. But it's best to avoid this motivation to stay hydrated if your relationship with your body is already complex. Just to throw it in there, research does back these claims. You should at least know that drinking at least 2 liters of water can help you burn more calories, but that's only something technical.

Instead, focus on other benefits. Getting enough water can prevent health problems such as kidney stones, which can form more easily if you're dehydrated. It can also prevent or treat constipation, which involves difficulty passing stool and bowel movements that are infrequent.

Water may also be able to prevent headaches. If you're already dealing with the daily stress of life, drinking enough water can help treat headaches that are sometimes caused by dehydration. One caveat is that the types of headaches you get matter.

If you decide to drink alcohol, drinking water can prevent hangovers, as alcohol is known to dehydrate you. Studies also show that even mild dehydration may have an effect on your moods. As such, drinking water may be able to help you feel better.

8. Keep a food diary

Food journaling is often hailed as the perfect way to help anyone who wants to change their goals around food. There's something else that happens to you when you decide to write something down.

Some experts even go as far as suggesting that you track your moods along with your food intake. A food diary may work for you if you have a hard time remembering what you ate that day. Binge eating also involves mindless or distracted eating, as such, thinking about what you eat will force you to slow down a bit.

When you keep this food diary, it helps just to write down what you ate without judging yourself. Your goal isn't to keep a diet, count calories, or keep up with a plan. That comes later, and with time. Keeping track of your moods when you eat may also force you to identify triggers. Research shows that using this simple tool could actually cut down on binge eating. You can use a pen and notebook, or an app.

9. Volunteer!

Binge eating and the guilt that it causes you may rob you of feeling good about a variety of things. Why would volunteering help you? First of all, it connects you to something you care about without having food involved. Most importantly, it can help you reclaim your life and time by providing you with an outlet to help others.

The benefits of volunteering have been found so beneficial that many programs that help people with eating disorders include this as part of their services. Binge eating can cause a person to feel depressed, and volunteering is a great way to combat these issues.

Many volunteers learn new skills, share their passions, and make new friends. Research also shows that volunteering can recuperate a sense of purpose, and it can even help students with their future and academic endeavors. Many organizations accept volunteers on a rolling basis, and you can even keep trying until you find the cause that calls you.

10.   Practice watching movies and TV without food

On March 2013, Harvard Medical School published an article discussing why distraction can lead you to overeat. Part of this is that you're multitasking, which makes you more likely to eat faster or stop paying attention to your eating patterns.

The study concludes that this is because attention and memory can have an impact on how you eat every day. Your brain gets the signal that you're full about 20 minutes after eating. That means if you eat too fast you may end up too full, and you're more likely to eat quickly if you're simply not paying attention to what you're doing.

Distraction means that your meal doesn't get stored in your brain's memory. If your brain doesn't remember you just ate, it simply won't register the food. This makes it easier to continue with eating behaviors that make you binge eat.

Chapter 12

Do You Suffer from Emotional Eating?

O besity levels amongst people are certainly higher than they have ever been in history. This trend has spread throughout the world. People are gaining weight at excessive rates. But the big question is, why? What is it that is really causing people to gain weight?

The quick answer is to blame it on the junk food, and that would be the logical answer. There are so many food manufacturing companies that are creating junk foods which are not healthy for people to consume.

Junk foods are basically processed foods that have been altered from their natural state. The common junk foods contain added pesticides, preservatives, flavorings, sugars, salts, seasonings and all kinds of things that are bad for our health.

Unnatural foods will cause you to feel unnatural. In other words, they will cause you to feel symptoms of stress, anxiety, irritation, irregular heart beat and more.

Even though these symptoms may be natural in some life circumstances, when they are caused simply by food then they are unnatural.

The Real Reason

We know junk food is the problem for most health problems in America and other developed countries. Until government agencies ban junk foods from being sold in the supermarkets, they are always going to be there and people will always buy them.

It is no surprise to ordinary citizens that junk food is bad for them when they see it in the supermarkets. They know cookies, cakes, pizza, and fried foods are just going to make them feel lousy after they eat them. But they continue to eat these foods anyway. So again, why?

The real reason has to do with stress more than anything else. People live such stressful lives in the modern age. They have to worry about making a living, taking care of their kids and so on. It gets to a point where they really have no time to relax and feel comfortable at all.

People in stressful situations tend to form bad habits in order to relieve their stress. One of the biggest habits people develop is binge eating on junk food.

Once this happens, the unnatural chemicals and additives in those foods will raise their stress levels even higher. So instead of treating the problem, junk food just makes it worse.

Control the Eating

It is important that you understand the difference between emotional eating and regular eating. For example, if you are on a strict diet and you are able to control what you eat, this is regular eating.

When someone eats to relieve their stress and anxiety, this is emotional eating. Even someone who regularly sticks to a healthy diet regime could find themselves eating poorly if they are stressed. This is the inner demon that you must learn to fight.

So, how does someone gain the discipline to control their eating under stressful situations? The first step is to try and distance you from all unhealthy foods.

This means no filling your kitchen cupboards with junk food from the supermarket. Only fill your house with healthy foods. After all, if there are no healthy foods in your house then you won't be tempted to cheat.

Now if you are away from your house, like at work, then you might find vending machines nearby that will tempt you into eating poorly. These are always hard to resist for someone under distress.

Fortunately, there are certain types of foods you can eat beforehand that will help limit your cravings to relieve stress pains.

Avocados – These are fruits that contain folic acid and vitamin B6. These nutrients have been scientifically proven to reduce stress levels by helping the central nervous system function well. It also contains potassium, which regulates blood pressure.

Salmon – This type of fish is very high in omega-3 fatty acids, which can elevate you into a good mood. These acids also keep your heart strong, especially if your cortisol levels are high. These stress hormones get released under pressure and cause damage to your heart if they remain high. Omega-3s will prevent this.

Broccoli – This vegetable is a good source of Vitamin C, which is what strengthens the immune system. When you feel stress and anxiety, it can put a burden on your immune system. It will even make you susceptible to colds and flu bugs.

Almonds – These nuts are loaded with magnesium, which is a mineral that lowers cortisol levels. This will calm down the nervous system when it starts feeling stressed out. You will even sleep better as a result of eating these, which will then help you in other ways as well.

These are the four foods you should always have on hand with you, whether you are at work, school or wherever.

Two of these foods are so simple to carry that you don't even need to cook them.

As for the salmon and broccoli, just cook them beforehand and then bring them with you in a Tupperware container.

Now, every time you start feeling stressed out during the day, go ahead and eat a little bit of these foods. You don't necessarily have to eat bites from all of them, although that wouldn't hurt. If you are under time constraints and don't have time to eat, then almonds would be the best food to munch on.

Almonds are hard food and can conveniently be eaten from your desk at work or anywhere. Since they lower cortisol levels, this will ultimately be what you need to keep your stress under control. Then when you have your next lunch break, go ahead and eat the rest of the foods to calm yourself further down.

Now you can still eat other fruits and vegetables if these mood friendly foods don't fill you up. But just remember to stay away from all processed foods because they will reverse the positive feelings you have already endured from the healthier mood foods.

Eventually, you will start to develop a habit of controlling your mood through healthy eating every time you feel stressed out. Then it will become a routine for you, which means you will have successfully turned a bad habit into a good one.

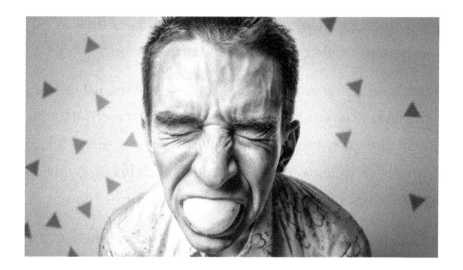

Chapter 13

Emotions Are Linked to

Your Eating Attitude

E very individual that is struggling with emotional eating has an underlying reason for the habit. We can say these people are eating their feelings even though they do not know. Eating is a combination of pleasure and addressing body needs. If these two things cannot happen together, then it means one will always supplement the other. If you do not feel like eating, because you do not find pleasure in it, then you have to eat for the sake of your body. Your body needs the energy to carry out its normal functions. Similarly, if you are not hungry but you cannot resist eating, then you will be eating to derive pleasure from it. This latter scenario is what emotional eating entails. Eating not because it benefits your body but because it merely makes you feel good. The desire to feel good is caused by a variety of reasons, negative ones in most cases.

Body Hate and Insecurity

The eating habits of most people are influenced by a predetermined attitude that includes how the food will affect their bodies. This is mostly seen in people that are either underweight or overweight. The former will, in most cases, eat too much food thinking it will help them gain some weight. The latter will go to the extent of starving themselves in their desperation to lose a few pounds. All these people end up harming themselves due to insecurity and discomfort with their bodies. Once you start complaining about your body, your attitude towards food will likely be affected by your desired physical results rather than overall health benefits. A simpler way of dealing with your body is to accept your body. Trying to look for an ideal body will only put unnecessary pressure on your eating. What other people think about your body does not matter, provided you are comfortable with it. Many people, including those close to you, will come up with ideas about how you should look. You can take in all those opinions but decide for yourself at the end of the day.

Stress and Anxiety

Just like in the case of weight, stress, and anxiety can induce in you weird eating habits that include overeating and under-eating. This happens when you do not find an effective way of dealing with stress. Constantly eating because you are stressed has the same effect as alcohol. You will eat all you want, but when the food is digested and assimilated, your stress or anxiety will come back, maybe with an even higher intensity. The food you eat because you think it will reduce stress is not normally healthy and balanced. A careful observation of such eating habits shows the kind of food that is eaten by the individual is mostly junk food, and the eating itself is irregular. The other aspect of eating habits related to stress is eating less than the recommended amount or starving yourself. This is already a disaster before arrival. This is not only bad for your body health; it can also worsen your stress and anxiety level. Either way, you will always be alternating between a starvation/binge eating and stress.

Too Much Excitement

From the surface, excitement is a good feeling which everyone would want to experience. However, too much of it is poisonous like everything else. Have you ever received the very good news that made you leave plate full on the table? Does this happen every time you are feeling happy? If that is the case, then you almost have an eating disorder. A disorder where your emotions affect the way you eat. The best way to handle this weakness is by giving yourself time to tame your excitement before you begin eating. If your excitement is the kind that makes you forget your meals entirely, create a timetable for all your meals, and ensure you follow it religiously. If you happen to trip to the new arrangement, always try to compensate for it as soon as possible. The key here is to maintain a regular eating pattern irrespective of your mood.

Deprivation and Cravings

This is a challenge, especially for people struggling with dieting. Sometimes the limitations of the types of food you eat are overwhelming. It is at this point that an individual starts eating emotionally. One thing I strongly believe in when it comes to food is the fact that we can always replace a certain type of food that is out of our reach. If you feel deprived of a certain cereal because your diet does not allow, remember there are many more cereals you can choose from. Cravings can be tamed by finding replacements, as well. However, if the desire to eat a particular food becomes too strong, you can improvise by playing mind games with that emotion. Simply include that food component in your meal but in a much-regulated manner. Throw in a bar of chocolate in your shopping bag if you feel you cannot beat back the craving. Make the chocolate come last when you sit down to eat. It will motivate you to eat the rest of your food to satisfaction. Curing that craving that moment will keep you going for a couple of days or weeks. However, it could turn out to be a risky adventure as this act of 'appeasement' might transform into a habit you cannot stop. In case you notice that the craving does not seem to go away, look for a more effective way of dealing with it. You can decide to suppress those thoughts altogether, refuse to think about it at all costs.

Anger

It is quite easy to notice when anger is affecting you're eating. Most people tend to eat very fast when they are angry. Some eat slowly and sometimes end up forgetting there is a plate in front of them. These two types of people are exhibiting poor eating habits. An aggressive eater has two problems; they won't be able to chew their food properly, and this greatly interferes with digestion. They are also at risk of eating more than they need. This does not only pose a problem for their digestion, but it will also affect the person's eating pattern. Once you notice that you are bitter or angry, postpone all your meals until that feeling has receded. However, if the problem does not seem to go away as fast as you expect, at least try to concentrate on your food. Pay attention to every meal and every bite in particular. If you try to enjoy your food, you will start feeling happy. The anger will have reduced or ended completely by the time you finish it. This will affect positively on your eating because you will be finding comfort in food whenever you get angry. However, anger should not be a motivating factor that enables you to take your meals.

Sadness

This is another emotion that you need to monitor as far as your eating is concerned. It is difficult to prevent ourselves from being sad, but we must not allow it to get into the way of our eating. A typical sad moment is when we have lost a loved one.

It is when food is nowhere near the top of our list of priorities. There are rare cases where sadness induces a huge appetite. You should always remember that food helps us to deal with our emotional distress. The food has to be in the right proportion and taken in the right interval. Again, concentration is all that is required to make sure your eating is not affected by the prevailing mood. Observe how the food behaves in your mouth, feel the taste very bite you take until it is no more. Feel your teeth sink into the food, notice how your molars crush the huge chunks into small pieces. Notice how your tongue turns and manipulates food in your mouth before pushing it down the food pipe. Do this for every bite until the plate is empty. You can also apply preventive measures to ensure your meals are not affected when you are sad. Ensure there are no stressors around mealtimes. In modern error, the use of mobile phones has facilitated a swift transfer of information without mentioning the role they play when it comes to social media. One sad call or text message is enough to spoil your entire appetite at the dining table. This is the reason some people, especially families, have banned the use of mobile phones during meals. You never know what you will see immediately you open your social media account, let that phone be until you are done eating. It will shield you from potentially sad information.

Fear

Fear is one emotion that has the potential of paralyzing you completely, including your eating pattern. Normally, eating is part of the treatment for fear. It gives you the energy needed to think properly and even overcome fear. However, there are cases where the fear itself is brought about by the food, a condition known as cibophobia. This fear is sometimes specific to a certain type of food or group of foods, such as undercooked foods. This condition can interfere with your entire eating habits if not handled properly. If you find yourself vomiting just because you have seen a certain food, it means you have a serious problem with your eating that needs to be addressed. Some people are also afraid of cooking their food, another kind of fear known as mageirocophobia. This is a dangerous kind of phobia in that it makes you completely dependent on bought foods or those cooked by other people. This means that if you are not in a position to buy food and there is no one to give it to you, then you run the risk of starving. It also means you will have irregular eating patterns since you are not in control of all your meals.

Self-esteem Issues

Some people find it hard to eat properly in the company of other people. This kind of individuals normally ends up eating less than they should. If you have this problem, you ought to address it immediately because you might not always avoid people. A good way of handling issues with self-esteem when it comes to eating is by forgetting everyone else around you when it comes to meals. This does not mean you forget your manners too. Enjoy your meal decently, concentrating on every bit of it. Feel how your body is responding to the food. Do you feel satisfied or do you need some more? Don't feel shy if you are not satisfied; ask for more until you are full. If it is a buffet, fill up the plate with your favorite food without minding who is watching. The only thing you need to mind is the food will be enough for everyone; otherwise, do not leave that place with a half-full stomach. Do these things every time you are eating with a group of people, and your self-esteem will cease to be a barrier to healthy eating habits.

Chapter 14

Relationships and Eating

Child, family, stress and eating

Children with inadequate eating practices are more probable to become overweight or underweight. It seems to have become an increasingly prevalent practice today. Poor dietary habits often result from an unnecessary consumption of electricity and insufficient use of micronutrients. Although poor eating practices can only be a component of the cause, they contribute considerably to the danger of obesity and malnutrition. This can set the phase for more negative health issues (e.g., heart and liver illness), particularly if bad dietary habits are prolonged to adulthood.

While some of the issues that caused, you're eating problem may root in the childhood and the way in which you were brought up, that doesn't mean that your family is a bad influence to stay away from. On the contrary. You can use the adult relationships that you have with your family members to be emotionally mature and overcome the burdens that you've been carrying on your back. The role of your familiar circle isn't just to support you through weight loss. You can share your insights with them, and reach out to voice your deepest needs, forgive, and heal from old trauma.

With stress-eating, you are eating for two reasons. The first reason is to calm yourself down, and the second reason is to recover from the loss of energy that happened during the stressful episode. Either way, using this, you can find some coping strategies to address your stress instead of ignoring it. Here are the steps to recover from stress-eating:

·   The first step to prevent stress eating is to learn how to recognize your triggers. To do this, keep a journal and note situations when you feel like you want to eat for other reasons than being physically hungry.

·   Next, you want to track your behaviors. This will give you insight into your eating habits. When tracking your hunger or eating behaviors. Include the intensity and the fluctuations of your hunger. You can rate them on a scale of 1 to 10, to compare the intensity of different triggers.

·   Also, note the particular activity that you are doing, and whether it is, in any way, unpleasant or annoying.

·   Write down the descriptions of feeling physical sensations, and thoughts that come into your mind.

·   Start thinking about the ways you can calm yourself without food. Think about other activities that calm you down that you can do instead of eating. Can you listen to music, meditate, read a book, or do yoga? Can you make certain lifestyle changes that will allow more time for rest? If your problem seems to be too difficult to handle on your own, you can always talk to a therapist.

Stress eating can also have a lot to do with your early childhood development. If your parents used food to calm you down instead of teaching you how to process your emotions, you might have learned that the best way to be calm in adult life is by eating.

Another reason that you might be stress-eating is that you have difficulty acknowledging your own feelings. When you have negative feelings, you want to remove or destroy them. This can leave lead to unhealthy behaviors because feelings don't go away when we want them to. You can suppress them, but they will reappear sooner or later.

So, what can you do to stop this? The solution is to break the cycle, discover your personal stress triggers, and find the best ways to cope. You will do this by listing the current influences that are making you feel stressed out. You can do this by sectioning different areas of your life, or by laying out only the most important influences. Here's a small task list to help you out:

· Write down all the symptoms of stress that you are currently experiencing.

·   Sort them by physical, emotional, and psychological.

·   After this, it is time to rediscover the ways in which you were using food to cope with stress.

·   List the foods that you enjoy eating while you are under stress. Note the amount of food you are eating, and how you feel before and after eating it.

·   What do you hope to gain by eating in a stressful situation?

Creating this list of personal insights is a good way for you to figure out how your mind and body choose to cope with stress.

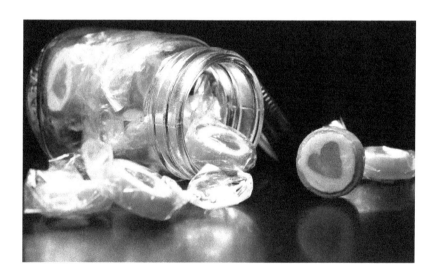

Chapter 15

Mindful Eating

Mindfulness is a simple concept that states that you must be aware of and present in the moment. Often, our thoughts tend to wander, and we might lose track of the present moment. Maybe you are preoccupied with something that happened or are wondering about something that might happen. When you do this, you tend to lose track of the present. Mindful eating is a practice of being conscious of what and when you eat. It is about enjoying the meal you eat while showing some restraint. Mindful eating is a technique that can help you overcome emotional eating. Not just that, it will teach you to enjoy your food and start making healthy choices. As with any other skill, mindful eating also takes a while to inculcate, but once you do, you will notice a positive change in your attitude toward food.

Reflection

Before you start eating, take a minute and reflect upon how and what you are feeling. Are you experiencing hunger? Are you feeling stressed? Are you bored or sad? What are your wants and what do you need? Try to differentiate between these two concepts. Once you are done reflecting for a moment, you Acan now choose what you want to eat, if you do want to eat and how you want to eat.

Sit Down

It might save some time if you eat while you are working or while traveling to work. Regardless of what it is, you must ensure that you sit down and eat your meal. Please don't eat on the go, instead set a couple of minutes aside for your mealtime. You will not be able to appreciate the food you are eating if you are trying to multitask. It can also be quite difficult to keep track of all the food you eat when you are eating on the go.

No Gadgets

If all your attention is focused on the TV, your laptop or anything else that comes with a screen, it is unlikely that you will be able to concentrate on the meal that you are eating. In fact, when your mind is distracted, you tend to indulge in mindless eating. So, limit your distractions or eliminate them if you want to practice mindful eating.

Portion your Food

Don't eat straight out of a container, a bag or a box. When you do this, it becomes rather difficult to keep track of the portions you eat, and you might overindulge without even being aware of it. Not just that, you will never learn to appreciate the food you are eating if you keep doing this.

Small Plates

We are all visual beings. So, if you see less, your urge to eat will also decrease. It is a good idea to start using small plates when you are eating. You can always go back for a second helping, but this is a simple way to regulate the quantity of food you keep wolfing down.

Be Grateful

Before you dig into your food, take a moment and be grateful for all the labor and effort that went into providing the meal you are about to eat. Acknowledge the fact that you are lucky to have the meal you do, and this will help create a positive relationship with food.

Chewing

It is advised that you must chew each bite of food at least thirty times before you swallow it. It might sound tedious, but make it a point to chew your food at least ten times before you swallow. Take this time to appreciate the flavors, textures and the taste of the food you are eating. Apart from this, when you thoroughly chew the food before swallowing, it helps with better digestion and absorption of food.

Clean Plate

You don't have to eat everything that you serve in your plate. I am not suggesting that you must waste food. If you have overfilled your plate, don't overstuff yourself. You must eat only what your body needs and not more than that. So, start with small portions and ask for more helpings. Overstuffing yourself will not do you any good, and it is equivalent to mindless eating.

Prevent Overeating

It is important to have well-balanced meals daily. You shouldn't skip any meals, but it doesn't mean that you should overeat. Eat only when you feel hungry and don't eat otherwise. Here are a couple of simple things you can do to avoid overeating. Learn to eat slowly. It isn't a new concept, but not many of us follow it. We are always in a rush these days. Take a moment and slow down. Take a sip of water after every couple of bites and chew your food thoroughly before you gulp it down. Don't just mindlessly eat and learn to enjoy the food you eat. Concentrate on the different textures, tastes, and flavors of the food you eat. Learn to savor every bite you eat and make it an enjoyable experience. Make your first-bit count and let it satisfy your taste buds. Now is the time to let your inner gourmet chef out! Use a smaller plate while you eat, and you can easily control your portions. Stay away from foods that are rich in calories and wouldn't satiate your hunger. Fill yourself up with foods that can satisfy your hunger and make you feel full for longer. If you have a big bowl of salad, you will feel fuller than you would if you have a small bag of chips. The calorie intake might be the same for both these things, but the hunger you will feel afterward differs. The idea is to fill yourself up with healthy foods before you think about junk food. While you eat, make sure that you turn off all electronic gadgets. You tend to lose track of the food you eat while you watch TV.

Chapter 16

Tricks to Help Manage Binge-Eating

H ere are some daily tricks and tips you can use to help prevent falling off the wagon.

Steer Clear of Diet Fads

Multiple studies have proven that when you are compelled to avoid certain types of food, your cravings and binge-eating urges increase. And all types of diets have some kinds of foods in their exclusion list.

Therefore, steer clear of all diet fads, and simply focus your entire attention on healthy small portions of healthy and nutritious foods of all kinds. You will have better control over your cravings.

Do Not Skip Meals

Skipping meals tends to increase your hunger pangs, which have a direct impact on cravings, which, in turn, could result in overeating. Studies have shown that eating one large meal each day instead of 3-4 small meals resulted in increased blood-sugar levels and the levels of ghrelin, the hunger-stimulating hormones.

Both these biological elements contribute significantly to binge-eating. Therefore, avoid skipping meals. Moreover, scientists have observed through various studies that people who start the day with a healthy, nutritious breakfast tend to have reduced ghrelin (the hunger-stimulating hormone) activity, which, in turn, results in lowered cravings.

Get Sufficient Sleep

Although this point has been made earlier too, it makes sense to include it in the daily tips because the lack of sleep has been directly connected to binge-eating as proven by many studies conducted by different experts in the medical field.

Eat Mindfully

When you eat slowly and mindfully, being aware of every emotion, feeling, taste, and other aspect of eating, you will be more aware of when you are feeling full which will help you stop eating. Mindful eating improves eating behaviors.

Get Physical Activity

Include a walk/run/gym regimen into your everyday routine. Many studies have revealed that binge-eating disorders are reduced significantly by increased physical activity. Additionally, physical activity has proven to enhance moods and reduce stress thereby preventing and decreasing emotional eating.

Drink Plenty of Water

Studies have proven that individuals who drinks plenty of water decreases their food consumption as compared to those who do not stay well-hydrated. Drinking water has been observed to boost metabolism and help in weight loss. Staying hydrated is critical to controlling your binge-eating behavior.

Include Plenty of Fiber in Your Daily Meals

Fiber reduces hunger pangs by moving slowly within the digestive tract, and also by keeping us feeling satiated for a sustained period of time. Scientific studies have shown increased fiber intake in daily meals reduces hunger pangs, calorie intake, and increases satiety.

Practice Yoga

Yoga is an ancient health-boosting technique that has exercises and postures designed to align and harmonize the workings of the body and mind. Studies have proven time and again that daily practice of yoga reduces cravings and helps you manage emotional eating problems.

Don't Forget to Update Your Journals

The importance of maintaining a journal for your binge-eating problem has already been stressed. Do not forget to update your food and mood journals on a daily basis. The entries made here will be the cornerstone of the success of your endeavor to get rid of the binge-eating disorder from your life.

Follow these daily tips and tricks unfailingly. Don't worry excessively about relapses. They are bound to happen. Get back on track and keep up your fight. Sustained victory has more to do with persistence and patient effort rather than occasional on and off blitzkrieg flashes.

Conclusion

Binge-eating occurs when an individual consumes a large quantity of food rapidly in response to specific emotional triggers rather than genuine hunger. Simply overeating is not enough to qualify you as a binge-eater though; everyone overeats once in a while. Instead, the way you eat is only an indication of a much deeper problem in the interaction between you and food. Binge-eating is a physical, biochemical, and psychological disorder all at once. A binge-eater typically gets attracted to food when he is on a binge. This seemingly uncontrollable physical attraction leads to a change in the biochemistry of the body and leaves a psychological deficit to be made up.

Binge-eating it though occurs most commonly as a part of two eating disorders; Binge Eating Disorder (B.E.D) and bulimia nervosa.

That means frequent episodes of binge-eating characterize BED. Bulimia Nervosa shares the same core principles with BED except that people suffering from Bulimia Nervosa get so distraught after bingeing that they attempt to purge the food they have just eaten out of their system. They may try to do this via a variety of ways. Some sufferers engage in marathon fasts, hoping to get rid of the food they have eaten or as atonement for binge-eating. Others may choose to induce vomiting to get rid of the food they just ate, or engage laxatives and diuretics to rid themselves of the wet weight of the food they consumed. It is even possible for chronic sufferers to participate in a strenuous, overboard exercise in the belief that it burns off the excess food they have eaten. Unfortunately, these all cause more damage than help.

They may choose excessive fasting, vomiting, laxatives, diuretics, or excessive exercise to get rid of the food they have consumed. We can consider Bulimia Nervosa a form of BED with the added attempt to get rid of the food that one consumes. Since you understand this already, I may use the term "binge-eating" interchangeably in this text. Just bear in mind that BED is differentiated from Bulimia Nervosa by attempts to purge.

Now, just how common is binge-eating? The stats speak for themselves. 3.5% of Adult American women and 2% of American men suffer from binge eating disorder while this figure may be as high as 16% in adolescents. Again, two-thirds of people with BED are overweight and actively trying to reduce their weight. That shows that BED is a real threat when it comes to nutrition in the 21st century.

Unfortunately, many people fail to understand that binge-eating can be a psychological disorder. Many people have embarked on weight-loss crusades lasting several months and even years, without any noticeable difference, all thanks to the fact that they binge-eat a lot. It is relatively common to find an individual who claims that he loves food a lot and can eat a mountain even when he is not hungry. Such a person might have "BED" without knowing it. As we will discuss later, binge-eating may even be the root cause of some of the social and health problems you are battling. Also, Binge-eating isn't just about the quantity of food that an individual consumes at a sitting, it is about how it gets eaten too; secretive, too rapid and too frequently. All these contribute to providing the ill-effects of binge-eating.

CPSIA information can be obtained
at www.ICGtesting.com
Printed in the USA
BVHW091507220621
610211BV00004B/897